Photographs – back cover

These photographs, together with a series of annotated photographs that show the history of the development of the lesion, can also be viewed at: **www.lentigomalignamelanoma.info**

i **4 August 2011**
two days after diagnostic biopsy: stitched wound

ii **29 September 2011**
immediately prior to first plastic surgery

iii **early October 2011**
after plastic surgery 1: stitched wound covered with steri-strips

iv **7 October 2011**
eight days after plastic surgery 1: supportive taping, after removal of stitches

v **late October 2011**
scar from plastic surgery 1 is healing well

vi **5 November 2011**
two days after plastic surgery 2: stitched wound covered with flesh-coloured steri-strips

vii **13 November 2011**
ten days after plastic surgery 2, and two days after removal of stitches and application of supportive taping

viii **13 November 2011**
taping removed: scar visible, healing well

ix **4 December 2011**
scar – 4+ weeks after plastic surgery 2

Foreword

This book is not intended to be a source of medical advice. If material in this book gives rise to any concern about your own health, professional medical advice should be sought.

Anyone who notices an unusual skin lesion or blemish should seek advice from qualified medical staff. Such professionals are very willing to help by offering appropriate reassurance or by referring the patient to a specialist. I have heard many doctors say that they would rather be approached than have a situation where a patient runs the risk of not bringing a problematic lesion for treatment.

Annotated photographs demonstrating the history of the development of my lesion can be viewed at www.lentigomalignamelanoma.info

The book cover photographs, which show stages of treatment of the lesion, can be viewed at the same site.

Introduction

The lesion known as lentigo maligna melanoma accounts for approximately twenty per cent of all malignant melanomas. It occurs mainly in older people.

After plastic surgery for the removal of my own lesion, I decided that it might be useful to write an account of my experience – from the first appearance of brown markings on my face, and onwards, until the scarring from the necessary surgical interventions began to settle down.

Being an amateur photographer, my husband has always used pictures to document family events, and my troubles were no exception. He took photographs at the time of the diagnostic biopsy, and then continued to add to his collection as events unfolded. From this sequence I have selected the photographs that appear on the back cover of this book. My husband and I have also looked through photographs from the family collection, and have identified a sequence that shows the appearance of the first 'freckle' in 1997, and its gradual extension over the years, which led to the development of the lentigo maligna melanoma. All these photographs can be viewed at www.lentigomalignamelanoma.info

It had soon become obvious to me that these lesions are not easy to recognise. Many well-qualified medical professionals who had seen me in a variety of contexts had not noticed the existence of mine. Once I had the definitive diagnosis, whenever possible I offered to let doctors and ancillary staff see the lesion 'in the flesh', as I felt that this was a way in which I could help.

When I realised that the presence of an atypical lesion, largely in people who are near or beyond retiring age, was unlikely to lead to a patient writing about it, I became determined to make my account widely available. Since then, several NHS personnel in senior posts have encouraged me to do this, saying that, whatever the diagnosed condition, any such writings by patients are hard to find.

Any person facing a surgical procedure necessary for his or her health is likely to experience some intense emotional states at times. The impact of the diagnosis, the intrinsic uncertainties, repeated visits to hospital, and the waiting times, are some of the many challenging aspects of such situations, and can lead to anxiety and distress of varying levels. It is not uncommon for patients to describe this as feeling that they are 'living in a parallel universe'. In my writing, my intention has been to indicate areas of emotional stress without describing them in particular detail, as I felt that in general that approach would be the most appropriate.

Each person is different, and I am in a position where I can represent only my own experience. However, I do believe that many people who have been through similar hospital procedures will be able to identify with parts of what I have described, and I hope that those who are waiting may draw strength from my story.

It is my sincere wish that as well as being of some support and encouragement to people in difficult times, this book will lead to a wider awareness of the existence of this particular kind of lesion.

Background

I am fair-skinned and my eyes are grey. I am nearly sixty-four years old. I was born in Birmingham. My father and his family were from there, and my mother was from Yorkshire.

As a child, when the sun was hot I used to hide in the shade. When the sun was very hot, I used to feel ill, even in the shade. In the summer holidays, my mother let me go to bed in the heat of the day, and I stayed up in the evenings, when it was not so hot.

When I went to secondary school, the girls in the 'in crowd' used to sunbathe, and their skin would burn and peel. As they sat chatting to one another they would tug at flakes of peeling skin, and compare the burnt areas on each other's backs. I could never understand why they did this. It might eventually have led to the development of the coveted tanned appearance, but the thought of lying exposed to the burning heat of the full sun was something I could never imagine being able to endure, and I never tried it. As a result I could feel rather left out.

As an adolescent I became interested in agriculture – dairy farming in particular. The sheds and milking parlours were invariably shady and cool. Cold water was readily available from a long hosepipe, and whenever hot weather became too much for me, I could simply turn the hose on myself. Invariably my clothing consisted of jeans and a lumberjack-style check shirt, sleeves rolled up to just below my elbows. I never worked in agriculture for extended periods of time. The longest was fifteen months, and these times were spread over about ten years – later years being employed in agricultural research, which took place largely indoors.

I have never worn skimpy clothing. I could never understand why people wore things that seemed to have no value either for protection from the bright sun or from cold weather. Consequently I have never owned a sleeveless top, a garment with a plunge neckline, or a short skirt.

When my friends and neighbours are sitting out in the sun, I am in my house, or I find a shady spot outside. The rooms at the back of my home face almost due north, and therefore hardly ever get the sun. This suits me very well. In the summer I can be certain of safety from the effects of strong heat and light, and in the winter, the warmth of the weakened sunlight is welcome at the front of the house.

Of course, there have been times when I have had to be out in the direct sun. I have always found such days to be a trial, and am greatly relieved when summer, with its risk of hot days, is past.

I have observed over the years that more and more people travel abroad for holidays, in search of the sun. I show a friendly interest in such perceived pleasures, but I would never inflict such torture upon myself.

Travelling twenty-five miles to the sea on a calm overcast day to swim in the deliciously cold water is a delight to me. It brings me great happiness. I do like walking – preferably through shady woodlands. Rain makes me feel safe.

The first sign

When I was about 50 years old, I noticed the sudden appearance of a lightish brown mark a short distance above the level of my left eyebrow. Its presence annoyed me, and I used one or two creams to try to 'fade' it or otherwise modify its visual impact. Its sudden appearance puzzled me. I had never taken an interest in makeup, and I soon found that attempting to camouflage it was more annoying than the mark itself.

At some stage I remembered that I had a read an article that had made a link between certain metabolic processes and such marks, but I couldn't locate the article, and in any case I knew that the category of dietary deficiency that was quoted was not relevant in my case. In fact, I didn't fit into any category of faulty diet. My training in agriculture and nutrition had resulted in my acquiring an extensive knowledge of sensible dietary choices – food types and their origins being of appropriate concern to me.

No one commented on the existence of the brown mark. It seemed that I was the only person who was aware of it.

Progression, and a basal cell carcinoma

Several years later, it was as if the mark divided into two. There was still a mark in the original site, but a similar one appeared, below it, although not exactly, and not far away from it.

I didn't like this. Still no one commented on the brown marking. It was as if to everyone else it didn't exist. Yet to me it was definitely there, and I didn't want it to be. I discounted any idea of asking for help from the NHS, as I imagined it would be viewed as a cosmetic problem. I concluded that I would just have to continue to put up with it.

The brown marks remained, apparently unchanged.

Not long before my daughter's wedding, more than four years ago, I noticed a small red mark on my right temple. I took little notice of it, as I assumed that it would go away again quite quickly.

The day of the wedding approached, and still it was there. I asked my daughter to get rid of it for me, as I didn't want it to appear on the wedding photos.

She examined it. 'It doesn't look like the kind of thing you can squeeze,' she decided. So I had to leave it there. In my mind it constituted another 'cosmetic' problem, and was therefore not a medical issue.

The following spring I went to see my GP about another matter. While I was there, I pointed to the red mark, which by then was larger. As I did not think I could ask for help with it, I simply asked what it was. To my surprise, the GP referred me to the local minor surgery unit.

There was a delay before I was seen there. I remember waiting trustingly, believing that I would eventually hear something. However, under increasing pressure from friends and family, I made enquiries, and it became apparent that the referral had been lost from the system. When I became aware of this, I insisted that steps were taken to ensure that this did not happen to anyone else. I remember saying to someone at the time 'How awful it would have been if a little old lady was sitting in her house patiently waiting for her appointment, while a malignant melanoma was growing on her face.'

Eventually the day of my appointment came. The doctor asked me about the history of the red mark, examined it, and then told me that it was too big for him to remove. I felt quite shocked. He then went on to say that he thought it was a basal cell carcinoma and that he would take a punch biopsy. He also said that he would refer me to the hospital dermatology department.

The biopsy confirmed the doctor's diagnosis. I was seen at the dermatology department, where the lesion was measured and photographed. Then a date was set for its removal, together with an adequate margin of healthy tissue around it.

As I waited for that day, I found out as much as I could about such lesions. I had been told that it had been caused by sun damage – by ultraviolet light (UVA) – to the deeper layer of the skin. How on earth could that be so in my case? I wondered. But then I learned that such damage could take place even as a result of being out and about on relatively overcast days. Apparently, just the very act of being outside regularly over years – following pursuits such as walking, golfing and gardening – was sufficient. I wasn't a golfer, but I did like being outside, so long as it wasn't too sunny.

I was told that now I had developed one of these lesions, I might well develop another. I learned that once the tumour begins to form, it takes about two years for it to show on the surface of the skin as a small mark – red in my case. If left, such lesions can adhere to the skull, and are then more complicated to remove. I was lucky, as

4

mine had not reached that stage.

An elipse of skin was to be removed – horizontally – by a very experienced doctor. I was told that the scar from this would fade into the lines of my forehead.

When I presented myself on the appointed day, I was directed to lie down on an examination couch. My face was covered with a large sheet of paper that had a hole in it to allow access to my right temple. The surgeon told me to shut my eyes. I remember feeling helped by the fact that he was cheerful and pleasant. He injected local anaesthetic around the site, waited, and then checked that I felt the area to be numb.

After that I felt what seemed to be two thuds on my forehead, as the elipse of skin was removed. I smelled burning flesh as the wound was cauterised, and then it was stitched closed. In addition the wound was covered with what were referred to as 'paper stitches'. I didn't know what that meant until I saw them later, in a mirror. A nurse gave me instructions about the care of the wound and when to see the GP practice nurse for the stitches to be removed.

I like to think that I managed to walk out of the room 'normally'. The surgeon was standing at a small table in the corridor outside. I shook his hand and thanked him. His handshake was firm and connecting. It wasn't good that I had developed a basal cell carcinoma, but I felt lucky to have had a good person to remove it.

Walking across the courtyard outside with my husband, I thought I was going to be sick and faint. I told myself firmly that I was having a normal reaction and that I was going to cope with it okay.

During this necessary contact with the dermatology department, it had never occurred to me to ask anything about the area above my left eyebrow, although by then it was even more obvious. After all, in my mind it was just a cosmetic problem. The real worry had been the basal cell carcinoma on my right temple, and its diagnosis and treatment had been a significant challenge for me. Now it had been removed, I didn't need to worry about it any more.

No one at the dermatology department had commented on the brown bits of skin near my left eyebrow. It was still the case that nobody at all ever commented on it. It was always as if it didn't exist – although of course I could see it. I didn't like it being there, but I just had to put up with it.

I still have the passport-sized photographs that I needed when I applied for my bus pass, and I can see the presence of both the basal cell carcinoma on my right temple and the brown markings above my left eyebrow.

At some stage the main upper section of the brown marked area seemed to fade considerably. I felt uplifted. Maybe the whole thing would now begin to disappear. I could still see the faint outline of that faded upper section, but the brown in it was almost invisible.

However, this year, I felt quite upset when I noticed that the part that interfaced with my eyebrow was darker than before, and the brown colour had returned to the 'faded' upper part. I was going to have to struggle harder to ignore it! I had never been a person who looked in the mirror very often. Maybe I should just not look in the mirror at all…

The diagnosis

All through my life, midges have demonstrated that they like feeding from me, so it was no surprise when I found myself scratching yet another midge bite on the back of my upper right arm. My husband and I were driving off for a weekend away, and I was relaxing at the thought of pleasant times ahead.

I pulled the flesh of my arm round so that I could see the midge bite… and then I froze. What I had been scratching was a mole with a dark centre. I felt paralysed. I couldn't say anything about it.

I pretended my way through the weekend, and when I returned home I looked on reputable websites for photographs of moles. I learned that the one I had corresponded to a group that should be monitored, as they had a higher risk than ordinary moles of becoming malignant. Reassured by this information, I went to my GP practice and showed the mole to a locum doctor, who referred me to the hospital dermatology department.

By great good fortune, this doctor pointed to the brown marks on my forehead, and asked me what they were.

'I've had them for years,' I replied casually. After all, this was the NHS, and cosmetic surgery wouldn't be available... I didn't want to ask if they could be removed only to hear the word 'no'. I have a sense that there is something about the word that for me signifies more than its actual meaning at the time, and this can often hold me back. I have never really got the bottom of quite why that is the case.

When I left the practice I resolved that I would ask at the dermatology department what the marks were. I reasoned that since a GP had commented on them it would be all right for me to mention them.

I was seen at the dermatology department less than three weeks later. Its new appointments system allowed me to be fitted in quickly, as my work schedule could be adapted to free up time at short notice. I was pleased about this.

I sat in the large open waiting area, and waited for my turn to come. Many posters on the wall informed any reader of the dangers of sunburn. I read them with interest, knowing that there was never any chance of sunburn for me – now or in the past. For me it was no hardship at all to avoid intense sunlight. I thought how awful it must be to develop dangerous skin cancer from sun damage.

I was ushered into a consulting room by a male doctor with a friendly professional manner. He examined the mole on my arm, and what he told me corresponded exactly with what I had learned from the internet sites.

I thanked him, and then, pointing to the brown marks on my

forehead, asked, 'Could you tell me what this is?'

He examined the area through the same instrument as he had used on the mole.

'I'll get someone else to take a look at this,' he told me quickly, in careful tones.

He disappeared from the room and returned a minute or two later with his consultant, a woman. She examined the mole, confirmed his view, and said that it would have to be monitored, or removed. I opted for removal, and was told that this would be arranged. Then she looked at my forehead.

'Can you stay on today so that we can photograph it and take a biopsy?' she asked in the same carefully normal tone as her colleague. 'We'll see you again in four weeks.'

'I put plenty of money in the parking meter,' I said, helpfully.

She continued. 'The area is too big for us to deal with, but we can refer you to the plastic surgeons and they can tidy it up for you.'

She left, and the male doctor filled in some forms, asking me a number of questions as he did so. I told him that I was grateful for their help, and added that my sister-in-law nearly lost one of her legs as a result of a malignant melanoma. He asked me not to speak while he concentrated on filling in the rest of the form, and I fell silent.

The female consultant had seemed so kind. I wondered why that was. I hadn't imagined that I would be offered any help with this. Plastic surgery? If indeed I was later referred, what would it involve…?

The photographs were taken in a different part of the department, and then I returned to queue for the biopsy to be taken. Ignorant of what I was facing, I sat and read one of the newspapers.

A young Chinese doctor took a substantial biopsy from the darkest part of the brown marks. She was working under the supervision of a fully qualified doctor, and it was quite interesting to hear them talking about what they were doing and about other medical subjects. I found the procedure rather challenging, as the site was so near to my eye, and I hadn't been prepared for this. I had only come to have the mole on my arm examined.

When the procedure had been completed, I was given instructions for the care of the stitched wound, and was told when to see the GP practice nurse for removal of the stitches. As I turned into the corridor, I encountered the female consultant and saw that she was standing beside the man who had removed the elipse of skin from my forehead more than three years earlier. I was certain that the woman was looking at me compassionately. Why was that?

Feeling quite shaky after the excision of the biopsy, I did my best to smile. Pointing to her companion, I said in my best 'upbeat' way, 'This is the man who took a chunk out of my forehead three years ago.'

Outwardly stable and inwardly tottering a little, I made my way out into the open air. I told myself firmly that surely I must have imagined the compassionate look on the consultant's face. Instead I decided that she must be intrinsically a pleasant person. I made my way to my car, phoned my husband to tell him about the biopsy, and then sat and gathered myself until I was certain that I was fit to drive.

The next day I learned from my next-door neighbour that her childminder's husband was dying from invasive malignant melanoma. Apparently, he had seen his GP some months earlier about his concerns about a mole on his back, but the GP had said that there was nothing wrong. I felt awful for him. What a dreadful situation. That poor man...

The removal of the stitches was uneventful, and I applied Kamillosan ointment to the biopsy site regularly, to keep it moist while it was healing. It also protected it whenever I was swimming in the sea.

Not long after that one of my best friends fell over backwards in his flat and hurt his neck. At the age of ninety-two, this interfered with his mobility, and he fell several more times. The necessity of helping him as much as I could completely eclipsed any thoughts or concerns I might have had about my biopsy.

Just over three weeks after my visit to the dermatology department, I received a letter from the woman consultant to say that she had been trying to phone me. How strange... I read on. 'Very early stages of skin cancer...' What exactly did that mean? I read more. 'After plastic surgery it should not require complicated treatment such as chemotherapy...' My legs suddenly felt weak, and I had to sit down.

My husband looked through the letter and thought that it was reassuring. I wasn't convinced. My daughter and I were to spend the afternoon together as we had planned to swim in the sea. I showed her the letter, and she immediately offered to come with me to my next appointment with this consultant – which by then was only a few days away. I felt very grateful, and accepted.

I prepared a list of questions in advance of the appointment. The first was to ascertain whether or not I had a malignant melanoma in and above my left eyebrow.

Before I set off for that appointment, the postman delivered a letter that gave me details of when and where I would meet the plastic surgeon. That appointment was only three days away. This certainly was good news. In my churned up state, I was glad that I did not have to wait long.

A few hours later the dermatology consultant confirmed that the biopsy had revealed the presence of malignant melanoma.

'I thought that it was always associated with moles,' I said.

'About fifty per cent of them aren't,' she explained.

How was it that this vital piece of information had evaded my awareness all these years? When I was in my early twenties I had read an account of a case of malignant melanoma that had developed in a mole. It had almost killed the sufferer. Then, sixteen years ago I had heard that my sister-in-law had one in a mole near her ankle. A friend's sister had had one in a similar position. No one I knew had ever spoken of one that was not in a mole, and I had never seen any literature about non-mole melanomas.

I went through my list of questions. I wanted to know how deeply the melanoma had penetrated. Here the news was good. The penetration in the biopsy was in the category of less than 0.5 mm, for which I learned that the prognosis is excellent. I then asked what the clear margins around the biopsy had been. The consultant looked puzzled.

'What do you mean?' she asked in an ordinary way. She waited for a moment before adding gently 'The biopsy was taken from the centre of the affected area.'

From the time when I set off for this appointment I had been controlling my feelings very carefully, but now I had to stop feeling anything at all in order to be able to cope with the rest of dialogue. I felt quite unsteady.

Further discussion revealed she expected that when the rest of the area was removed, some cancer cells would be found, although to a lesser depth. I asked whether there would be some longer-term monitoring once the treatment was over. She told me that I would have two or three appointments at the plastic surgery department after the necessary surgery, and then I would be referred back to her department, where I would be monitored for a minimum of two years.

She checked my lymph glands, and looked for moles on the parts of my body that I could not see for myself. She commented that I had only a few moles, and I remember feeling that this was a good thing. She checked the file to confirm that I was definitely on the waiting list to have the mole removed from my arm, but then surprised me by asking if I would like to have it off that day, if she could arrange it. I agreed without hesitation. The removal of that mole would be a big step in the right direction. It would mean that there was one less thing to worry about.

My daughter sat in the operating room while a trainee removed the mole under supervision. Again the dialogue between the doctors was very interesting. The only downside was that I was being cut again. The incision was deep enough that it required internal stitches as well as external ones. Before I left I was given instructions about how to care for the wound, and was told to have the external stitches removed by the GP practice nurse after five days. I learned that vigorous movement of that arm had to be avoided for eight weeks.

To have had my daughter sitting not far from where I was lying was a great support. And it meant that afterwards we were talking about an event that we had shared – which was quite different from trying to describe to someone what had taken place.

Plastic surgeons

The appointment with the plastic surgeon was not at the department of plastic surgery. It was at the cancer centre, which was at a different hospital. My husband couldn't find anywhere to park the car, so I went in on my own while he drove to on-street parking.

I did not have to wait long before I was taken into a room by a pleasant male doctor, who then spoke to me in such a compassionate way that I had great difficulty in preventing myself from crying.

He explained that because of the size of the area involved I would have to have a skin graft, and that this would be a full thickness one. He went on to estimate how much skin would be needed, and he examined the possible donor sites – behind my ear, behind my neck and above my clavicles. He thought that skin would have to be taken from the clavicle area to yield a large enough piece and that would be a good enough match for my face. Amongst other things he told me that the malignant melanoma had invaded hair follicles in my eyebrow, and that consequently most of my left eyebrow would have to be removed – so that I would be left with only a small section of it. He, too, checked my lymph glands.

Later, the consultant plastic surgeon joined us, and he was examining me when my husband arrived. To my horror, the consultant outlined an area of my face that was much larger than his younger colleague had indicated. He said that the site would require a centimetre clear margin round it, and that to ensure this he would need to harvest skin from the inside of my upper arm. He explained that in addition to removing much of the eyebrow and an area of skin above it, he would need to remove the skin between my eyelid and eyebrow. I felt terribly shocked, but did everything I could not to show it. I thought that if I showed anything at all, I might just fold up.

I learned that it is impossible to see where the margins of these lesions lie, even under the magnification used during surgery, and that only the laboratory report of the excised tissue would reveal the true picture. The consultant told me that if the lab finds there is not sufficient clear margin, he might be able to stretch an existing skin graft for one or possibly two places, but beyond that he would need to discard the graft and take another one. I was given the option of having the surgery done under general anaesthetic, but I declined, saying that I would have a local anaesthetic. I learned that I would be on the operating table for about an hour.

I asked when the surgery would be done, and was told that it would be in about two to four weeks' time.

Over the years, many people have commented upon the excellent quality of my skin. As my husband and I walked to the car, I sneered angrily at the memory of this. Then I realised that although some of it had been taken over by malignant melanoma, most of it had not, and the fact that my skin was of good quality would certainly be of help in whatever procedures had to be conducted.

A skin graft? The whole thing sounded awful... But what choice did I have? I supposed that there were other people, somewhere, who had had to have this done. My sister-in-law had had one on her leg, but I knew no one with one on the face.

I phoned each of our three adult children from the car, and each of them spontaneously told me that whatever the change in my appearance, I would still be the same person to them. I found this of comfort.

But exactly what would I look like after the surgery? I knew that I would not be able to hide the change, and this worried me. Friends reassured me that there would be cosmetic strategies that I could use to modify the impact of the scar and conceal the fact that I had only part of an eyebrow. They offered to teach me how to do it, once the scar had healed. It was very reassuring to know that there was a way out of my predicament.

When I phoned the GP practice at the beginning of the following week to make the appointment to see the nurse to have the stitches removed from my arm, I asked the receptionist if there were any staff who might like to have the opportunity to see the malignant melanoma on that day. I said I had picked up that it was a less common configuration. I then learned that the locum GP who had referred me to dermatology had a special interest in minor surgery. He later rang me, and I thanked him very sincerely for his input that had led me to finding the confidence to ask the dermatologists about the brown marks on my face.

Afterwards, various questions presented in my mind. What if I hadn't had the mole on my arm with a dark brown centre? What if I had had it, but hadn't noticed it? What if I hadn't gone to see that particular GP? What if he hadn't referred me to the dermatology department? The answers to those questions did not bear contemplating. I just felt extremely lucky.

Although the incidence of malignant melanoma is increasing, there are only around 1,200 new cases a year in Scotland, so it is important to offer to show diagnosed lesions to medical personnel. Being able to see one 'in the flesh' is much more effective than viewing only photographs. As I was having the stitches removed, two of the doctors and the senior nurse came to look at my face, and were grateful for having had that opportunity.

Before I left, the nurse confided that the consultant who was to operate on my face had rescued her from a very difficult medical situation a couple of years previously. I was very glad that she went on to tell me the details of this, as then I felt that I could trust him completely.

I rang my sister-in-law at the weekend. She was very kind to me, and talked the whole thing through.

'You *must* tell people,' she advised. 'I didn't tell my friends for weeks, and when they found out, they were angry with me. I told them that I couldn't just phone them and say, conversationally, "Hello, I've got a malignant melanoma." '

After that, neither of us could stop laughing.

I followed her advice, and gradually it became easier to talk about it.

I had noticed that the Macmillan cancer organisation had a helpline, so I rang it. There were a number of things that were worrying me – healing times of skin grafts, and levels of pain from the donor site and the grafted site. Since the plastic surgeon had said that he would have to cut the skin away above the eyelid, I wanted to know if this would disturb the functioning of the lachrymal gland. And would my eye have to be taped shut afterwards? I also began to wonder if I should ask to be given a sedative before the operation.

The nurse advisor said that my questions were entirely valid, and encouraged me to contact the surgeon about them. In the end I asked a district nurse friend my questions about skin grafts, and I wrote to the surgeon about the rest of them. I felt reassured when he sent a reply.

After about ten days, the wait for my date for surgery became very stressful. My attempts to obtain a more precise estimate of it came to nothing, and for a while I felt quite distraught.

During those difficult days an unexpected ray of sunshine arrived in the form of another letter from the dermatology department. It informed me that the mole which had been excised from my arm had been harmless – a 'compound melanocytic naevus'. Although harmless, I had no doubt at all that deciding to have it removed had been wise. In my position, the removal of a potential problem such as this had been entirely correct.

Then a letter arrived from the plastic surgery department with the date for my surgery. It was to take place almost exactly four weeks after I had seen the surgeon. As my husband was to be away from home with work responsibilities that could not be changed, our daughter promised to take the day off to be with me at the hospital.

During the waiting time, a friend put me in touch with one of her own friends – a homeopath who had had to have surgery on her face a few years earlier. I rang her, and she was very helpful – advising me to use arnica and calendula at a high potency. She told me where I could obtain these potencies, and I ordered them straight away. As I am experienced in the use of dowsing, I felt confident that I could use this skill to guide me about when to use these remedies.

Other friends wanted me to consider treating the cancer by alternative means. Although interested to hear about such approaches, I felt that I had no choice but to go ahead with the surgery. The melanoma was very near to my eye. I had lived a 'clean' life for decades, and I could not think of any extra lifestyle changes to adopt. I was certain that I could not afford to take the chance of delaying the well-proven treatment offered by mainstream medicine.

I was largely on my own for the four days before the day of the surgery. I was determined to make the best of those days that I possibly could. I swam in the sea, tidied my allotment, and went for a pleasant walk. I also made sure that the housework was up to date. I noticed that each day I spent some time in a kind of panic – sweating, and at times feeling that I was choking. I wasn't at all sure that I would manage to cope for an hour on the operating table, but I was determined to recruit all my inner resources to enable me to do this. I was certain that I didn't want the extra trauma of a general anaesthetic, and in any case I knew that it was fundamentally important to me to be fully aware of what was being done to me.

I felt fortunate that I had had my full eye check for that year only weeks earlier. However, because of ongoing irritation and disturbance in my left eye, the day before my date for surgery I asked an optician to check that eye for foreign bodies – particularly as I had had a bit of grit in it only days before. He found nothing, but gave

16

me useful advice about drops and ointments that might help.

I spent time in front of a mirror, using a reading lens to study the brown markings above my left eye, and reflecting on the fact that soon that area would look very different.

Plastic surgery

My daughter stayed with me overnight. I washed my hair in the evening, and when we got up the next morning, she went for a jog, and I went for a short walk. I noticed that my heartbeat suddenly began to behave very oddly, so I came straight back home, and we left for the hospital soon afterwards.

I found that sitting in the large day surgery waiting area was harrowing. I didn't know what to expect. Fortunately my daughter had brought some books with her and we spent some time discussing elements of her studies, which I found interesting.

After about an hour I was called for a brief preoperative check. The nurse told me that there had been two lengthy cases in theatre that morning. I asked if they had been emergencies, but was told that the patients had been on the standard waiting list. The nurse said that she imagined the surgeons would break for lunch, but after that I would be first on the afternoon list.

I had to wait for nearly two more hours before I was called to get changed. I was shown into what then felt like a cell and was instructed to remove all my clothing, except my pants, before putting on the clean gown that had been provided. The long wait had intensified my emotional stress, and I wished that I did not have to be on my own.

At last I was taken along a long corridor to a waiting room for theatre. The nurse was talking about how my particular surgeon usually arranged things, so I was entirely unprepared for what happened next.

I waited alone in that room for a while, and then a man I had never seen before came in, carrying my file with him. He was wearing theatre clothing. He introduced himself and told me that my case had now been transferred to the list of a different consultant. I tried to keep calm, but my legs suddenly felt extremely weak. I managed to say that I felt quite shocked by the sudden change. I was glad that he showed no sign of being defensive, and he explained that within the NHS, although continuity of care was preferable, it could not be assured. I said that I understood this, that I was not in any way trying to demand that the change was not made, and that I just needed to register the shock.

He assured me that he was very experienced in the kind of surgical procedure I needed. I was extremely grateful for the fact that he then sat and discussed my case with me at some length, leaving me in a position where I began to feel that he was a little less unfamiliar. He told me that I had a lentigo maligna melanoma, and that this kind accounted for around twenty per cent of all melanomas. I had never heard of this name before, and I asked him to write it down for me before I finally left. He said that once I had the skin graft on my face, the colour of it would always be different from the rest of my face. He also informed me that sometimes only part of a skin graft 'takes', and that this could be a problem. However, I learned that the donor site on my arm could be closed, and I felt very relieved to hear that.

My new consultant joined us for a while, and when he examined my face he said that it might be possible to avoid a skin graft. It was then decided that the damaged area would be excised, and only if the lax skin could not be dragged across sufficiently to close the wound would my arm be prepared to harvest skin for grafting. I also learned that I would be left with a little more eyebrow than I had thought – a third of it. He left, and the surgeon who was sitting with me gave me more information.

I remember signing the consent form that he handed to me and then saying 'We'd better just get on with it.' That was another moment which I have valued. I had been given a situation where it was I who initiated the final steps, and in my compromised state this was important to me. He left, and a nurse took me to the theatre in a chair with small wheels on it. Fleetingly I wished that this could be merely a rehearsal – like the day before getting married.

The nurse left me next to the operating table. Then I noticed that inanimate stationary objects in the room seemed to be moving, and I had to keep a very tight grip on myself to prevent this perception from engulfing me.

I have quite short legs, and the portable steps up to the operating table could not be found. I managed to climb on to the table – a manoeuvre which was applauded by theatre staff! The surgeon who had been sitting talking to me in the theatre waiting room conducted a more detailed examination of the site of the lesion. After that he went away for a while. I presumed that he had gone to discuss the situation with the consultant. Someone clipped a monitor on to my finger.

'Sorry to keep you waiting,' he said on his return.

A male nurse held my hand while the surgeon injected anaesthetic into my face – a procedure which I found very painful. My eyes had to be shut and covered, and my head was tied up to cover my hair. I thought that I could recognise the surgeon's voice, but I asked for confirmation so that I could be certain.

Lying on a table while a man takes slices off one's face is a challenging experience, but there are certain circumstances when this has to be endured, and this was one of them. I kept myself together by bringing into my mind all the people who had promised to think about me that afternoon, remembering what each had said to me.

Eventually the surgeon cauterised the blood vessels and closed the wound. I was aware that he had achieved this without the use of a skin graft. He then taped the wound with steri-strips. The pads were removed from my eyes, and he asked me to close my left eye. This action was difficult to achieve, but I managed to close the lid more than half way.

It was time to sit up, and a nurse stood beside me, ready to help. I declined her input, saying that I wanted to protect her back, and I demonstrated how tucking my flat hands – palms downwards – under my back at the upper part of my pelvis, thus tilting it, allowed me to sit up without effort.

Somehow I managed to get back into the wheeled chair, and I waited there while the surgeon wrote up his notes. He made a note for me of the name of the melanoma, together with his own name and that of the consultant, and handed it to me. We shook hands, and I was taken away to the recovery area. Prone unconscious figures were being wheeled along converging corridors to the same destination. I had no doubt at all that for me it had been right to avoid general anaesthesia for this procedure.

Later, in the changing room, I managed to get my clothes back on and then went to find the nurse, who was filling in a discharge sheet. She gave me some verbal instructions about how to manage the wound site – including advice about using ice, covered in a clean tea towel, as already a 'black eye' was forming. She added that she didn't know how I'd managed to have the procedure done under local anaesthetic – a comment which I valued.

I had the presence of mind to ask for a contact phone number to ring for advice if I encountered any problems during the first 24 hours, and I was given the number of the plastic surgery ward. I found this very reassuring. It meant that if necessary I could speak directly to people who were experienced in the treatment of this kind of wound.

My daughter was waiting for me in the 'departure lounge', and we left promptly. I was desperate to get out of the hospital before I started reacting to what I'd endured. I was profoundly grateful that I did not have a skin graft and that I still had a third of my eyebrow, but I felt in a state of shock. My daughter commented that I looked a lot better than she had feared.

At home she stayed with me. She brought everything that I needed, and she kept telling me not to lean my head forward, as had been advised by the discharge nurse. My husband returned in the evening. However, not long after he left to drive our daughter back to her flat, the wound began to bleed profusely. At first I didn't know what to do, but then I remembered that the nurse had said something about pressing a clean pad on it if it bled. A clean pad? What could I use? I managed to find an old muslin nappy, and pressed it hard on the wound.

Very tired by now, I went upstairs, covered the bed in dustsheets, and put a clean red towel handy. My daughter had already arranged several pillows for me so that I could sleep propped up, as I had been told at the hospital. Somehow I managed to clean my teeth without leaning my head forward. In bed, the wound bled again. I felt very undermined by this, but glad to have my muslin nappy to hand. I clutched it all night, applying it whenever I felt anything wet on my face.

Recovery

The next morning my husband departed again for work, but it would only be a few hours before one of our sons was due to arrive to sit with me. I positioned myself carefully on a suitable chair, leaned back, and waited. I was plagued with worry about my left eye. I was gradually getting used to the unpleasant sensation of the whole area being 'trussed up', and although the eye was not shutting properly, this difficulty seemed a bit more manageable. But there was a gremlin at work inside me that was saying 'Remember all the disturbance you've had in that eye for more than a year. There were all those sensations of there being bits in your eye when there weren't... And those distorted eyelashes in the outer corner that you pulled out one by one many weeks ago. Maybe the melanoma caused all of that.' I reminded myself that a senior eye surgeon had examined both my eyes only four months previously because of the presence of a vitreous detachment. Yet this did nothing to allay my fears, as he had said nothing about the melanoma – which must have been clearly visible to him then.

When my son arrived, I told him what I was worrying about, and we agreed that I would tell the hospital staff at my next appointment.

He went to the GP practice and collected my prescription for pain relief, and then we sat and chatted about many things. It was good to spend those hours with him.

The next few days went by in a bit of a blur. I often had a headache, or at least an unfamiliar feeling in my head that felt like the aftermath of being kicked down the street. The vision in my left eye was disturbed, and remained so for far longer than the discharge nurse had indicated. I noticed some distortion of the skin just above my eyelid – as if it was tugging diagonally – but the surgeon had warned me to expect things like this, so it wasn't a surprise and did not alarm me.

Every night I slept with my bedroom window open. This helped with the struggle my eye was having with dryness. I was profoundly grateful for the fact that since the price of petrol had increased so much, almost all the boy racers who had frequented the road outside at any time of the day or night had disappeared.

Conducting my life without leaning my head forward was tricky, but not impossible. I had no doubt in my mind how important it was to make sure I did this. If I forgot, even for a minute, I could feel pressure build up in my face and the wound quickly felt more uncomfortable.

I felt exhausted, and could fold up completely with little or no warning. But gradually I gained strength, and began to go out for short walks near my home. I managed to make myself go to the local post office, and was greeted kindly.

I noticed that some car drivers stared at me strangely as they passed along the road. When I was feeling upbeat I could think 'Yes, have a good look. It might be you next month.' But if I was feeling low, it hurt.

I felt that I was making real progress when I managed to wash my hair – taking care to keep the wound dry.

After eight days, I returned to the hospital to have the stitches removed. I could not imagine quite how that would be achieved. It seemed to me that the steri-strips were more or less welded in place by congealed blood, and I felt a grating anxiety about the prospect of the procedure.

The staff nurse was wonderful. She talked to me for a while about what I had been going through, and explained why my head had been feeling so strange and my eyesight disturbed. She said that blood would have pooled in the eye socket, and that this would have put pressure on my whole head. As I grasped the meaning of what she said, I found it very helpful. After that, I believed that, given time, the distortion in my vision would improve.

Then she asked me to lie back, and she worked on the wound slowly and carefully until she could remove the steri-strips and then the twelve stitches. This hurt only a couple of times. She said that the wound was healing very well, and I told her about the homeopathic remedies that I had been dowsing each day, and using when indicated.

When she had finished, she put small strips at right angles along the wound to support it for a few more days. I was glad of this, and I was also relieved that it was less exposed to view than it otherwise would have been. I wasn't really ready yet to face the full impact of the scar and how others would react to it. I thought that I must look as if I had been 'bottled' in pub brawl, and as a non-drinker I found this upsetting. My eyelid was dragged up a bit more because of the new taping, and although this was unpleasant I did believe that the problem would slowly settle down.

My last appointment at the hospital was to be in five more weeks' time. The nurse had assured me that in cases like mine it was only a small number of people who needed to have further work done.

I was keen to get the laboratory report as soon as it became available. I left a letter at my GP practice about this, as each surgeon I had spoken to had said that, once available, doctors could access it electronically. I did not want to have to wait until my final appointment at the hospital before hearing the results.

When the time came, removing the supportive strips was not as tricky as I had imagined. I took them off one by one over a period of about 24 hours.

Later, when most of the scabs had fallen off, it became very obvious that I now had a piece of eyebrow that was at right angles to the rest of what remained. A friend said that I looked like an owl, and found it rather endearing, but to me it was yet another thing to trouble me, at least at first.

As time went on, what surprised me was the number of people who did not notice that I had a considerable scar and an absence of two-thirds of my eyebrow. I could only surmise that people were engaging with my personality and not the appearance of my face, and I slowly began to draw comfort from that.

Time passed, and I heard nothing about the lab report. I started to feel overwhelmed with the stress of waiting, and had a headache with a sore neck for much of each day. Then I woke up one morning with my heart beating very strangely. This went on for hours and hours every day. A friend ordered me to go and get it checked.

The hospital doctor at the out of hours unit was very thorough. After organising a range of tests and checks, he referred me to another unit for further tests at a later date. I found all this very helpful, and although my heart did not begin to settle down until many days later, my alarm at its very disturbed beat was reduced.

It was Wednesday afternoon, almost four weeks after the surgery, and there was still no sign of the lab report. I had finished my work for the day, and I decided to spend some time trying to tidy our garage – in an attempt to do something useful that might also distract my mind from its uncomfortable preoccupation.

After a couple of hours I heard the phone ringing, but I left it, knowing that I would not be able to reach it before it switched to the callminder. Nearly an hour passed before I decided to check to see if a message had been left. I imagined that the caller had been a friend or a family member.

The message was indistinct, but I could make out the name of the hospital where the surgery had been carried out and a phone number – which I rang straight away. The caller had been the consultant's secretary. She said that I wasn't to worry, but the lab report had revealed that I needed further work done on my face. She went on to say that this could be carried out the following week if I could attend then. I said straight away that I could be available on that date, but added that I needed to know exactly what was to be done. She told me that the consultant would phone me at the end of the following day.

My husband wisely suggested that we arranged to see the consultant at that time, so I rang back, and the secretary was able to arrange it. Driving to the hospital the next day, I tried to guess what I would be told. Perhaps there were a couple of places where the required clear margin had not been achieved?

I learned from the consultant that the whole area had to be re-excised, and that this decision had been taken at a team meeting. The healed scar was to be removed, together with tissue around it and at both ends – losing more eyebrow in the process. I was entirely unprepared for this revelation. I had never imagined that this would be the case, and instantly I re-activated the old familiar mechanism of detaching every one of my feelings from the situation, and conducting an entirely factual discussion. After all, I wanted to take in as much information as I could. In addition, I knew that it wouldn't be fair on the surgeon to have to witness outpourings of distress, and I felt that the more I could do to enable him to concentrate on his part of the overall task, the better the result was likely to be.

He told me that the melanoma can sometimes burrow under the skin. I learned that it can invade the eyelid – although he was able to reassure me that in my case this had not happened. I was very glad indeed to hear that. He said that if spreading, the melanoma would head for a lymph gland at the top front of where my ear joined my head. He stressed that if at all possible he would avoid the use of a skin graft, as he felt that on a face a graft was unlikely to look right. I learned that the depth of penetration in the tissue that had been taken out during the first surgery was consistently less than in the original biopsy.

He seemed certain that I would not be able to close my eye after the next surgical intervention, and said that drops could be provided. At some stage he had said that later I could have the line of the missing eyebrow tattooed.

He said that this kind of melanoma was often first commented upon by a friend or relative who had not seen the sufferer for several years. This certainly had not been the case with me. People I had seen in recent times had been a mixture of those whom I saw regularly or after long gaps. Even a local friend who is a nurse told me that despite the fact that earlier in her career she had seen a lot of cases of melanoma when she worked in the dermatology department, she had not noticed it on my face.

Before I left, he told me that he himself would be doing the surgery.

In the days that followed, I noticed that I had a fleeting impulse to phone my mother – who has been dead for nearly twenty years. After that came a few occasions when I wanted to speak to both my parents. My father died nearly thirty years ago. I could only surmise that I was near the edge of my ability to cope with what I was trying to face.

I concentrated determinedly on giving myself some good experiences. I swam in the sea, walked up a local hill, and did some sewing that I enjoyed.

My name

The Christian names that appear on my birth certificate are Alison and Mirabelle, but right from birth I have always been known to everyone by the second of these. This is not an uncommon situation, and I know quite a few people who have the same arrangement. Since the name Alison is only familiar to me when I see it written as part of my whole name, someone addressing me by that name is unlikely to get a response.

In the days when the NHS relied on paper records, the use of the name Mirabelle never presented any problem, but in the electronic age I have found that the NHS has increasingly used the name Alison, and I have had to correct that whenever necessary. However, of late, even that correction was not accepted, and in my currently very compromised state, I found that I was feeling more and more distressed by being consistently called by the wrong name, despite all my efforts to represent myself appropriately. I could not understand why this was such a problem within the NHS. I knew several people who had had no difficulty in ensuring the use of their correct name when it was not the first Christian name.

In desperation I contemplated removing Alison from my name in every context, and I spoke to my daughter, a lawyer, about this. She was startled, and when I explained what the problem was, she advised me that all I had to do was to find the right person in the NHS to correct it centrally. I felt supported by this, and began the task of discovering how to go about it. It took several telephone calls – being passed from office to office – before I found myself speaking to the right person.

I explained that not only was I finding the problem increasingly stressful, but also that there would be an issue if I were unconscious for some unforeseen reason and someone tried to elicit a response from me by calling me Alison. He acknowledged the sense of everything I was saying, and adapted the entry on the computer system for all hospitals straight away. He then advised me to write to my GP practice manager so that the records there could also be dealt with. Although I had already tried several times at the GP practice to have the problem resolved, I had never before written to the practice manager.

I drafted a letter that day, which I delivered by hand. The following week I was very glad to receive a prompt, helpful response from her.

There is no doubt in my mind that being called by the name with which I am familiar has made it less difficult to cope with my treatment.

Preparation for the further surgery

I made a GP appointment to talk about the impending surgery and the reason for it. I also wanted to mention the heart problem that had arisen.

The morning surgery was running quite late, but as it was a Monday morning, I did not think this to be unusual. However, when my time came, I found that the doctor appeared to be quite stressed. I was very glad that I had already phoned the local cancer support centre, and was to see someone there later that day. Perhaps that would be the best place to discuss my situation.

That appointment turned out to be entirely the right thing for me at that time. The person I saw was kind, balanced and well informed. She said that with the uncertainties inherent in my situation, she was not surprised that I was struggling. With my permission she later phoned the specialist nurse who was connected with both the dermatology and the plastic surgery department, and I spoke to her on the phone the next morning. She was able to explain a number of things in more detail. For example, I learned that my new scar would be at least twice as long as the one I already had. This was hard to hear, but I remember saying to her that I had already had to face the fact that I looked different, and that looking more different would not be such a big step. And I truly believed it.

The most precious thing of all that I gained from that conversation was that the nurse understood how stressful it would be waiting for the lab report after the next operation. She said that she would look out for it, and if I hadn't heard from her in two weeks after the surgery, I should phone her. She also said I could call her any time. Just to know that made an enormous difference.

Plastic surgery – 2

Examining my face in the bathroom mirror with a large magnifying glass in the evening before the day of my surgery, I saw a small, pigmented area not far from the inner end of the existing scar, and wondered if this was harbouring more melanoma cells. I was glad to have complete confidence that the consultant would do whatever he felt necessary.

The next morning I washed my hair as soon as I got up, and then went round the house, putting bottles of drinking water where it would be useful to me, and preparing my bed and also a place to lie downstairs. I put the phone number of the plastic surgery ward on the table in case I needed it after I got home.

Our elder son phoned. 'Be brave, Mum,' he said. I appreciated that call.

My husband and I arrived at the hospital in good time, and booked in at the day surgery waiting area. Having already been through this before, I was less anxious. I was familiar with the overall setup – the checks, the changing room, and the theatre waiting room. The prospect of not being able to close my eye after the surgery was not pleasant, but I had brought with me my collection of eye drops and ointments, and was determined to manage somehow.

The nurse who checked my blood pressure and filled in various forms was sympathetic to my need to be called by the right name. She was a student nurse, but as I noted her responses and demeanour, and the precision with which she went about her work, I imagined that her career would lead to her holding a responsible post.

The wait for my turn to get ready for theatre was a long one, and I did find it difficult. But then my name was called, and I went to get changed.

This time I was not alone in the theatre waiting room. There were two women already there, both about my age. Although a television was talking at us from the wall, we had an interesting conversation about general things, and I also learned that each of them was to have surgery on a finger. I was glad of the companionship, and even when one was taken away, the other woman and I were together until at last we were shepherded along the corridor to the next stage.

The nurse who took us on that journey recognised me from the previous time, and I told her briefly what was to be done. She looked uncomfortable, and I found this to be supportive, because I could see that she was contemplating what I was facing, and was finding it difficult.

The final checks complete, the consultant came to see me. He looked at my forehead again and we talked for a few minutes. He had certainly noticed the small pigmented area that I had seen in the bathroom mirror and said that he would have to remove it. He said again that I would lose more of my eyebrow. Then I signed the consent form, and he left.

Soon I was taken to the theatre in a chair on wheels. This theatre was different from the previous one. It was one of a whole corridor of theatres. I was wheeled through its anaesthetic area, and up to the table. This time there were steps for me to climb up.

Damp pads on my eyes. Hair covered up in a head wrap. Clip on my finger to monitor blood oxygenation levels. Body covered in what seemed to be a waterproof sheet. A nurse held my hand while the consultant's 'apprentice' injected my face with local anaesthetic. The nurse then stayed with me nearly all of the time.

I lay there, as motionless as I could possibly be, while the surgery was being carried out. My heartbeat was quite disturbed. I kept reminding myself that this was the one part of the normal reaction to being cut that my body was free to express. Being aware of the exposed flesh was something that I did not want to turn away from, but it was probably the most difficult part of all.

There was a time when the consultant's hand pressed quite hard on to my eyeball, and this was quite painful. I felt blood being mopped up, and also I knew when cauterisation was taking place.

During the time that my companion nurse was not apparent, my thoughts focused on how the consultant was certainly doing his best for me, and how he was trying to remove all the badness.

I heard clusters of words – 'want to avoid a skin graft', 'I'll take a little fat from underneath', and later, 'chlorhexidine, please', and 'I think this bit goes with that' (suturing the skin). There was another reference to the possibility of my tattooing the line of the eyebrow at a later date. One thing I found to be quite comforting was the way that towards the end of the procedure the consultant used my chest as an instrument shelf. This helped me to feel that we were doing something together, and that was important to me. I heard him ask for two different kinds of suture, and later for flesh-coloured steri-strips. His touch throughout was a little different from that of the previous surgeon. It was somehow slightly 'lighter' and more 'connecting'. Finally, a nurse did her best to wipe the blood away that had run into my hair by my left ear.

When it was time to sit up, I showed the nurse the same simple technique of tilting my pelvis as I had demonstrated to the previous theatre nurse, and again sat up unaided.

Before I was taken away to the recovery area, the consultant told me that I might have to have more tissue taken off later. He said that the melanoma can appear in 'islands'. I was interested to hear this from him. My husband had thought that the lab report's documentation of some small clear margins was promising, but I had felt that these might prove to be only gaps, and so I had been right about that. The consultant said that he would see me at his clinic in three weeks' time and that he hoped by then to have the lab report. He said he thought that the wound would not bleed, but that if it did, to use a clean pad, as before. He said that I would probably have a black eye. Then he shook my hand, and I was wheeled away.

In the recovery area I was shaking a lot, but otherwise okay. I thought that the shaking was a normal reaction to what I had endured, and did not try to stop it from happening. The mirror in the changing room revealed that the layers of flesh-coloured steri-strips had completely concealed most of the wound. All that was visible was the part that led down to the remaining small section of my eyebrow. Psychologically this was helpful. I wouldn't have to see the full impact until I returned to have the stitches taken out – and that was a whole week away. And stunningly, with a bit of effort I could nearly shut my eye!

The nurse gave me a discharge note and verbal instructions about my care of myself. I was not to lean forward or lie flat for four days. He offered to take the name bands off my wrists, but I just had to get away.

I cried and shook on the journey home. Again, I could allow myself this entirely normal reaction. There was a voice shouting in my head. 'I can't go through this ever again!'

Recovery – 2

Ice again. Homeopathic remedies again. I didn't bleed, and the predicted black eye didn't materialise! My eyelid was certainly dragged upwards tightly, but I was managing… And this time I was sure that it would gradually improve, as that is what had happened before. Also I knew that if I had to go through further surgery, I would. My left eye ran with tears in the night, but I could be confident that the wetness was not blood.

The next days were difficult. As before, I felt shaky and exhausted, but I was determined to be patient with myself, and I listened to Radio 3 at low volume. I couldn't read, as the balance of my eyes was disturbed – the left being distorted again. I often found myself lying with my right eye shut and the left open, as closing the left lid needed a special effort. I continued to sleep with my bedroom window open at night. The nights were colder now, so I wore more clothing in bed.

Examining the exposed part of the scar in the magnifying side of a shaving mirror, I made an amazing discovery. The stitches were a beautiful blue, which reminded me of the colour of feathers from kingfishers.

It was only now that our daughter confided that she was finding it quite difficult getting used to the sudden changes in the face that she knew so well. I told her I was very glad she had told me this, and had not kept it to herself any longer.

Day 5 came, and at last I felt that I could try to wash my hair. I made a small, water-resistant cover for the vulnerable area, and by that means I managed to keep water and shampoo away from it.

Out and about once again, I returned to the welcoming post office, and along the street I met people I knew. However, I did find that telling them a little of what had happened was almost too much. As more of the difficult feeling states that I had sidelined rushed to the surface, I could feel suddenly very weary.

Eight days after surgery, I returned to the hospital to have the stitches removed from the scar. The clinic was running late. A notice on the wall informed me that if a patient had to wait more than half an hour past the appointment time, someone would explain what the problem was, so the passage of time did not worry me.

Eventually, a senior nurse called for me. She removed the pink steri-strip structure and said that the scar was healing very well. This time there was a continuous suture and five individual stitches to be taken out. A student was present, and she asked if the eyebrow would grow back. The nurse told her that it could, but that in older people it sometimes didn't. I added that in my particular case it couldn't grow back because the skin containing the hair follicles had been removed. The nurse then placed strips of taping to support and protect my scar, and instructed me to go to my GP practice after a week to have them removed. Further instructions included how to massage the scar with E45 cream after that.

I was given an appointment for the consultant's clinic that was just over two weeks away. At that appointment the results of the next lab report would be discussed. I didn't have long to wait. My eyelid was pulling a bit more because of the taping, but I thought that, as before, this would settle down.

That night was difficult. My eye didn't feel right, and when I finally woke in the morning, it was extremely dry. I struggled with this through the day, and when I tried to read, I couldn't see properly from that eye, and there was a pronounced burning sensation. Eye drops didn't help, and I used some of the ointment that my optometrist had recommended. This helped the soreness and irritation, but my vision was very blurred.

I hoped that the following night would be easier, but I woke with severe pain that seemed to be coming directly from my eye. I noticed that there were plenty of tears, and I couldn't work out what was happening. Because of this I saw a GP the next day. By that time my eye and its surrounding tissues were very obviously inflamed. He examined me, and then phoned the plastic surgery department to discuss my situation. He felt that the supportive taping was dragging the tissues around the eye in a way that it could not cope with. He was advised to remove it, and was told that I would be given an appointment by the hospital for two days' time.

I was so glad the have that taping taken off. The relief I felt was almost immediate. On my way out of the building I noticed a woman staring at my face. For a moment I wondered why, and then I realised she was looking at the scar I had not yet seen. Sitting in the car with my husband, I looked at it in the mirror on the sun visor. I stared at it for a long time, realising that I had been waiting for the moment when I could see it. I had been fully present to the actions that had created it, I had felt the sensations from it over the days since, but without realising, I had been waiting to see it. Although it was longer than the previous one, and was branched at one end, the visual impact of it upon me was far less that when I first saw the one I'd had before. So I had been right – the biggest step had been the one from having no scar to accepting one being there, and the step up in size did not trouble me. I noticed, too, that I was pleased about the remaining piece of eyebrow. Although smaller, its presence was very welcome. And the 'owl' bit was no longer there.

After a few hours, my eye felt a lot better, and the following night my sleep was almost undisturbed.

The next day the specialist nurse who had promised to look out for the lab report rang me to see how I was getting on. I told her about the trouble I'd had with my eye, and that it hadn't been easy for me to make the decision to ask for help. She told me that I had done exactly the right thing, and was sympathetic about my finding myself in a situation which, already worrying, had had an extra concern added to it – something that on my own I could not understand. Speaking to her was again very helpful. In a week's time we would speak again, and by then she might have the lab report in front of her.

Soon after this conversation, I had a phone call from the hospital to give me an appointment to be seen there the following afternoon.

When I arrived there were quite a number of patients in the waiting area. I had assumed that my appointment was to see a nurse to have the taping redone, but I began to realise that this was a main clinic. As the doctors arrived, I recognised amongst them the man who had carried out the first surgery. Then I noticed one of the two men I had seen at my first plastic surgery appointment, and then the consultant who had operated on my face less than two weeks ago. Although there were a number of faces that I had not seen before, I found it surprisingly comforting to be in a place where three of the people who had been directly involved in helping me were present. I had known that they all worked closely together, but observing them around each other made that knowledge more concrete.

As it happened, I was seen by the first man from the initial plastic surgery assessment appointment. He examined me, and I talked to him about what had happened with my eye. I was greatly relieved to learn that the scar would not be re-taped. He said that it was healing very well and that I could now progress to washing my face, taking care only to pat that area dry. He had kindly checked to see if the lab report was available, even though it was rather too soon to expect it. Once more I heard that only the lab report would tell us if sufficient tissue had been removed, and that the melanoma could produce threads that spread where only the lab techniques could

35

detect. Before I left he told me to change the next appointment so that I would return after four weeks, not two, by which time the functioning of my eyelid could be assessed.

Several days passed. I was still quite tired, but was able to do more now. I went to a concert with my husband, and by chance a younger woman I had met at a concert some months previously arrived and sat in the seat in front of me. She asked me what had happened to my face, and when I told her, she confided that she had had breast cancer. She asked me if I was putting anything on the scar to aid the healing, and I told her what I had done so far. She encouraged me to consider putting vitamin E oil on it, saying that she had used it on her breast scars and had got a good result. She also knew of others who had used it successfully. I found this interesting, particularly as I knew that my sister-in-law had used vitamin E in a cream to help to heal the scars on her leg. However, I remembered that she could only do this later, and I made a mental note to ask her what length of time had elapsed before she could use it.

Waiting

In some ways, waiting for the lab report was not so difficult this time. After all, I knew more about what was involved, and consequently felt less at sea. I had heard from a friend that such laboratories aimed to have the reports ready within ten working days. I knew from what the specialist nurse had said that my tissue would have been marked 'urgent', and I knew from the doctor I had seen at the recent clinic appointment that the lab had to use special staining for such samples. And, of course, I was only too aware that the lab is always handling material from a very large number of cases.

I began to work again once I felt able to, and the days passed in a fairly ordinary kind of way. However, when lab-working-day fifteen arrived, still without any news, I knew that I would have to recruit more of my inner resources to focus my thoughts on other things in life, to ensure that difficult feelings did not engulf me.

I had already resumed my daily walk, and now I chose some piano music to practise. Playing a musical instrument can absorb all my concentration, and although I would never sit and play for hours, there is a very obvious after-effect, where my mind continues to be taken up with the sound of the music. I had completed the final section of a novella that I had begun to write some months ago, and I gave it to a few readers, inviting comments. I encountered other friends and neighbours – who were astonished at my news, as none of them had previously noticed anything amiss with my face.

I tried twice to contact the specialist nurse that week, but she must have been away, off sick or terribly overloaded with work. I could not guess what the lab report would reveal and how that would impact on my life, and I knew that I needed to know exactly what was in it.

At last the day came when I was able to speak to her, and when she read through the report she said she felt that no further work would be necessary. She told me that the relevant team meeting would take place in eleven days' time, which was four days before my next appointment at the hospital clinic.

Clinic appointment

To my profound relief, it was confirmed that no further surgery would be required. I also had the opportunity of discussing a number of points that I wanted to raise.

The tightness in the skin around my left eye was still quite pronounced, and continued to have an impact upon my eye. Although the acuity of vision had been improving, I still had problems with dryness, and the drops and ointment that had been recommended did not seem to help. Because of this I was by now very accustomed to sleeping with my bedroom window open.

Although the air in the middle of winter is very cold, I had adjusted to it, and certainly it made a big difference to the comfort of my eye.

The lymph nodes of my head and neck were checked. I was encouraged to keep massaging the scar with ointment, to keep the skin moist and supple. I was told that doing so would also help to resolve the pain that I was experiencing at one end of it.

I was asked to make an appointment to return in three months' time.

Now I knew for certain that I did not have to face any more surgery, in the days that followed my body began to express some of the shock reaction that it had held back, and I found myself crying and shaking. Although unpleasant, I had no doubt that this was a normal response.

A physiotherapist has since advised me how best to stretch the tight skin on my face. This will be a slow process, but eventually it should become easier to shut my eye. Meanwhile, the visual acuity of that eye has more or less returned to normal.

By now, five months had passed since I had found myself scratching that 'midge bite' on my right arm. The NHS had acted promptly and efficiently, and I was free to carry on with my life. Although I was to return to the clinic, I would no longer be dominated by a preoccupation with the unknown.

Some reflections

Alongside my interactions with health service staff, I found myself wondering what working life was like for each person in their particular area of responsibility. I was aware that they must have to cope with patients with a wide spectrum of varying needs – many of which were not necessarily obvious at first.

To the staff, the hospital building was familiar, as was the way it was run and also the faces of some of the people who worked there. Yet to many of the patients there was nothing that was familiar, and somehow they had to be helped through all the administrative and medical processes, in order to benefit from treatment.

How could a way be found which ensured that each patient understood whatever was necessary? I observed many interactions in which staff members persisted calmly and kindly until certain that a patient had grasped a particular message or piece of information. Whenever it came to my turn, I did my best to aim for a balance between expressing whatever was on my mind and trying to work out what was actually necessary that I should convey. I decided that I should err slightly on the side of saying more than I thought to be strictly necessary. After all, how could I be certain about what was, and what wasn't, essential to impart? Better to run the risk of sounding a bit ponderous than end up leaving out something significant.

In my earlier life I was involved in some medical research. When conducting a pilot study, I soon found that listening more broadly to what participants wanted to tell me resulted in our extending the range of relevant questions in the main study. This had confirmed to me my already established belief that there is always more to learn, and it helped me to find the confidence to ask for help and information when I needed it.

While being treated for the melanoma, it seemed to me that in the case of medical information there were certain previously agreed sets of facts that were repeated by different staff members whenever appropriate or possible. I thought that the consistency of delivery of such material was at times remarkable. Where there were variations, it gave me the opportunity to comment on this, and as a result I would often learn more of the background information, and I found this useful.

It was not only the training and expertise of each staff member that was important or apparent. There were many aspects of each personality that were clearly invaluable. The interfacing of these attributes and professionalism within teams and in direct contact with patients forms a cohesive web, without which the overall positive health results could not be obtained. That web is largely invisible, and is not easy to define, and yet it is a fundamental part. The bedrock of its substance depends entirely upon genuine expression of humanity. Perfection is not necessary. I would like staff to know that whatever their position in the hierarchy, each and every one of them is very precious to someone like me – a person who needed help with something that she could not achieve solely by her own efforts.

In quiet times in waiting areas, I would sometimes wonder about the distance each member of staff had travelled that day to get to work, and I wondered about the pattern of their shifts. I thought about their varying years of training and experience. However standardised the training, each person's work experience is unique, and therefore invaluable. Sometimes I had the opportunity to ask questions about all of this, and the answers were always of great interest to me.

The future

Not surprisingly, skin lesions impact upon my awareness in a different way from before. This is not just the case with my own body. I have found myself staring at the eyebrows of other people, often in a semi-conscious way.

Recently, after a phone call with an old school friend, I insisted that she went to her GP with an 'age spot' that she told me about.

'I'm sure it'll be all right,' she told me confidently. 'My mother had one in the same position.'

I was very forceful with her, insisting that she went to have it examined.

I do not think that I'll go ahead with tattooing to disguise the missing part of my eyebrow. I want to be able to check that area without anything getting in the way.

My consultant had reassured me that the distorted eyelashes that had worried me had nothing at all to do with the melanoma. However, I did not learn what had caused the distortions, and indeed continued to do so, until I visited a new optometrist some months later. When she had examined my eyes and the surrounding tissues very carefully, she told me that I was suffering from blepharitis, and that infection in the hair follicles was causing the growth of distorted eye lashes. She then gave me detailed advice about how to treat this.

* * * * *

Every one of us has to face something difficult. No one is immune from this simple truth.

Some resources

Cancer Research UK   www.cancerresearchuk.org

Macmillan Cancer Support   www.macmillan.org.uk

Changing Faces   www.changingfaces.org.uk

Let's Face It   www.lets-face-it.org.uk

Lightning Source UK Ltd.
Milton Keynes UK
UKOW051619120712

195897UK00001B/7/P